HAWTHORN

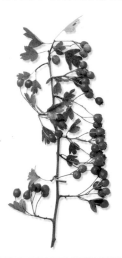

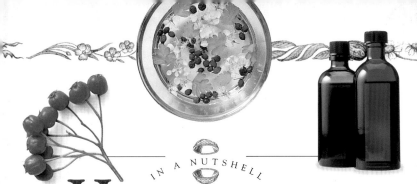

IN A NUTSHELL

HAWTHORN

CRATAEGUS MONOGYNA

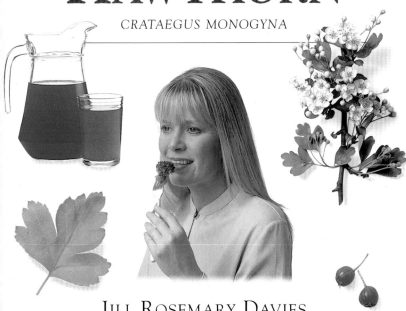

JILL ROSEMARY DAVIES

ELEMENT

SHAFTESBURY, DORSET • BOSTON, MASSACHUSETTS • MELBOURNE, VICTORIA

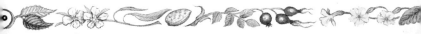

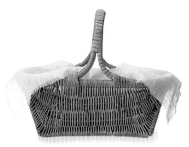

© Element Books Limited 2000

First published in Great Britain in 2000 by
ELEMENT BOOKS LIMITED
Shaftesbury, Dorset SP7 8BP

Published in the USA in 2000 by
ELEMENT BOOKS INC.
160 North Washington Street,
Boston MA 02114

Published in Australia in 2000 by
ELEMENT BOOKS LIMITED
and distributed by
Penguin Australia Ltd.
487 Maroondah Highway,
Ringwood, Victoria 3134

NOTE FROM THE PUBLISHER
Any information given in this book is not
intended to be taken as a replacement for
medical advice. Any person with a condition
requiring medical attention should consult
a qualified practitioner or therapist.

For growing and harvesting, calendar
information applies only to the northern
hemisphere (US zones 5–9).

Jill Rosemary Davies has asserted her right
under the Copyright, Designs, and Patents
Act, 1988, to be identified as Author of
this work.

Designed and created for Element Books with
The Bridgewater Book Company Ltd.

ELEMENT BOOKS LIMITED
Managing Editor Miranda Spicer
Senior Commissioning Editor Caro Ness
Project Editor Kate John
Group Production Director Clare Armstrong
Production Manager Stephanie Raggett
Production Controller Hannah Turner

THE BRIDGEWATER BOOK COMPANY
Art Director Rebecca Willis
Designer Jane Lanaway
DTP Designer Trudi Valter
Editorial Director Fiona Biggs
Project Editor Lorraine Turner
Photography Guy Ryecart
Illustrations Michael Courtney
Three-dimensional models Mark Jamieson
Picture research Lynda Marshall

Printed and bound in Portugal by
Printer Portuguesa.

Library of Congress Cataloging in
Publication data available

British Library Cataloguing in Publication
data available

ISBN 1 86204 557 7

The publishers wish to thank the
following for the use of pictures:
A–Z Botanical Collection: pp.7, 8, 9, 15,
48, 49b.
Bridgeman Art Library: pp. 10t, Rochdale
Art Gallery, Lancashire; 10b, Maas Gallery,
London; 13t, Christopher Wood Gallery,
London; 13b, Christie's Images, London.
E.T. Archive: p.11t.
Garden Picture Library: pp.22t, 23, 31b.
Image Bank: p.45.
Science Photo Library: pp.16, 18, 24.
Stock Market: p.27.

Contents

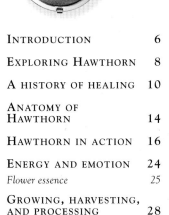

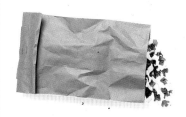

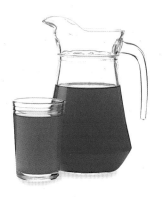

Introduction

IN WESTERN HERBALISM Hawthorn is the best-known herb for treating heart conditions and has also been used for a wide range of other medicinal purposes around the world.

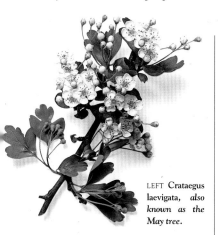

LEFT **Crataegus laevigata**, *also known as the May tree.*

Hawthorn is a dense tree with small sharp thorns. It can grow up to 33ft (10m) tall, and is often seen growing wild either as a lone tree or as ancient hedging.

There are over 1,000 different species and hybrids of Hawthorn throughout the world. The two species most commonly used for medicinal purposes in Western herbalism are *Crataegus oxyacantha* (now known as *Crataegus laevigata*) and *Crataegus monogyna*. This is because they contain the strongest quantity of Hawthorn chemical constituents and are widely available. They are fully interchangeable medicinally and share many of the same characteristics, as well as common names – for example, they are both referred to as English Hawthorn. In Eastern disciplines, both Chinese and Ayurvedic medicine use their own native medicinal species.

Crataegus laevigata is also known as Midland Hawthorn, or May. The Bread and Butter Tree is another name, derived from farmers' practice of nibbling on the leaves and flowers in order to take the edge off their hunger before breakfast. The oxygen that Hawthorn releases would have eliminated feelings of tiredness and dizziness and helped to ease yawning and general difficulty in waking up.

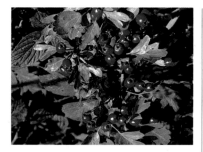

ABOVE *All parts of the Hawthorn "tops" are used medicinally – berries and leaves as depicted here, and also spring flowers.*

OTHER SPECIES

Crataegus laciniata – "Oriental Thorn"

This species is native to China and is planted in Europe as a very attractive ornamental tree. It has few thorns and grows to a height of 15–20ft (4.5–6m). The white flowers that appear in June are followed by deep-red fruit in the fall. The leaves are deeply cut and downy on both sides but especially on the underside.

Crataegus crus-galli – "Cockspur Thorn"

This species is native to central and eastern North America. It is often grown for its ornamental value or for hedging. The white flowers open in June and are produced in clusters that span up to 3in (7.5cm) wide. The leaves turn a beautiful scarlet in the fall. It has small fruit, which ripen in October and stay on the tree throughout the winter.

Crataegus pinnatifida – "Shan zha"

Shan zha is grown commercially for medicinal purposes. The berry is larger than European varieties: ½–1½in (1–3.5cm) in diameter.

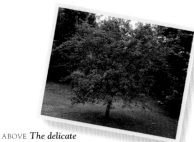

ABOVE *The delicate blossoms of Hawthorn burst into life in the spring.*

DEFINITION

The botanical name *Crataegus* comes from the Greek *kratos* meaning "hardness" (of the wood). The classification of the two most common species of Hawthorn also find their descriptive roots in the Greek: *oxyacantha* – *oxus* meaning "sharp" and *acantha* meaning "thorn" – and *monogyna* – *mono* meaning "one" and *gyna* meaning "female" (*monogyna* refers to its single carpel).

Exploring Hawthorn

NOW THAT HAWTHORN'S *healing abilities are becoming more widely recognised, more land is being given over to properly managed sustainable resource areas.*

WHERE TO FIND HAWTHORN

Hawthorn is a hardy shrub that grows in almost all temperate regions of the world. It can be found in Europe, North Africa, Western Asia, India, China, and North America, and was introduced to Tasmania and other parts of Australia by early British settlers. It prefers full sunlight but will tolerate most conditions.

Hawthorn is an aggressive settler on disturbed sites and consequently can often be found growing on abandoned fields and overgrazed pastureland, or on the periphery of hedgerows and forests. However, seedlings will rarely become established in pastures that are regularly grazed. Hawthorn is sometimes considered a nuisance, especially when it encroaches on farmland, because it can be tenacious and difficult to remove permanently.

In Britain and Germany during the period 450–1520CE, when farming was at its most widespread, Hawthorn was often laid to make hedging which,

BELOW *Hawthorn creates largely impenetrable hedges.*

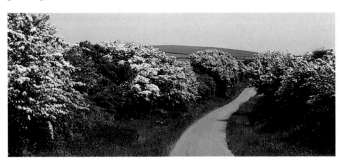

before the invention of modern fencing, was an excellent way of keeping farm animals in their fields. In Tasmania, Hawthorn hedges are considered to be part of the country's cultural heritage.

COMMERCIAL GROWERS

Because it is so prolific and easily obtainable, Hawthorn is not often grown commercially for medicinal use. Some areas where harvesting for commercial use does takes place have been designated "organic" or "wildcrafted" (see page 57), but usually these are long-established sites that have been claimed by commercial growers. Many of these areas are in National Parks in Europe, predominantly in Hungary, France, and Spain. The British and European Soil Association has set up a committee to encourage more wild and certified organic herb-collecting areas. France, Hungary, China, and India all export Hawthorn commercially. In the United States and Canada, commercial collection areas are in Oregon, Washington, and British Columbia.

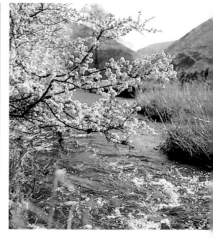

ABOVE *Hawthorn flourishes on the banks of streams and especially in chalky soil.*

SOIL REQUIREMENTS

Hawthorn appears to prefer alkaline soils and is very abundant in limestone areas. It will grow in almost any type of soil, but grows best in richer, well-drained soils, especially where water flows into ditches and streams; it is rarely found in wet peat and acid soils.

Hawthorn is a useful tree to grow in polluted urban areas, exposed sites, and coastal areas. The species C. *laevigata* can withstand temperatures as low as 5°F (-15°C).

A history of healing

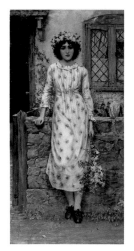

OVER THE CENTURIES, *a lot of folklore and traditions have grown up around the Hawthorn tree and, as with much folklore, they are sometimes contradictory. Hawthorn is, more often than not, seen as a tree that brings good luck to the owner and prosperity to the land where it stands.*

LEFT **The crowning of the May Queen with Hawthorn blossoms is an ancient tradition.**

According to legend, the god Thor created Hawthorn in a bolt of lightning. Because of this it was believed that Hawthorn would protect against lightning and storms at sea.

Traditionally, the Greeks and Romans used Hawthorn blossoms in wedding decorations to increase fertility and bring happiness. The Romans also believed that if you placed Hawthorn in babies' cradles it would protect them against evil. Both these traditions were carried over to England. In addition, the tree was thought to protect the house from evil spirits.

Hawthorn was the Sacred Tree of the sixth month for the Celts who called it "Utah," meaning "beauty," and the blossoms were used in the May Queen rituals. In the Middle Ages it was seen as a symbol of hope.

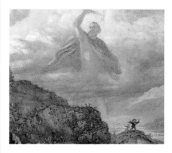

ABOVE *In legend, Hawthorn first sprouted after being thrown in a bolt of lightning by the god Thor.*

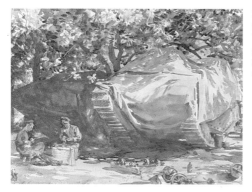

LEFT *Hawthorn helped the war effort during World War I, by providing substitutes for tea, coffee, and tobacco.*

The tree was once regarded as sacred, probably from a belief that the Crown of Thorns worn at the crucifixion of Christ was made from Hawthorn, and it was believed that placing a branch above the door would warn off negative forces. However, some people believed that Hawthorn's link to the crucifixion meant that it was a sign of bad luck and that bringing any part of the tree, especially the flowers, into the house would result in a death in the household.

The first Pilgrims emigrating to America named their boat *The Mayflower* after using Hawthorn wood to make some of the vessel.

Many Hawthorns grow to a great age as landmarks or boundary trees. There is a beautiful example at Hethel, near Norwich in England. When the tree was measured in the 18th century, it had a girth of 9ft (2.8m); it still stands but has now been reduced to a bush. The tree was called the "Witch of Hethel," possibly because of its curiously contorted branches. According to ancient folklore, it was thought that witches had the power to transform themselves into Hawthorn trees and that they held their rituals under Hawthorns.

During World War I, young Hawthorn leaves were used as a substitute for tea and tobacco, and the seeds were ground and used instead of coffee.

TRADITIONAL USES

Hawthorn was used to decorate the Maypole because the trees traditionally flowered on May Day.

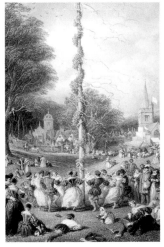

ABOVE *Maypoles were traditionally garlanded with Hawthorn blossoms.*

🌿 During midsummer festivities, Hawthorn trees were decorated with flowers and ribbons and people danced around them. Blossoms were strewn on paths.

🌿 Women believed that Hawthorn would keep them looking youthful.

🌿 Taking Hawthorn on fishing trips ensured a good catch.

Dioscorides, a Greek herbalist, used Hawthorn in the first century CE. In his writings he referred to it as *Crataegus Oxuakantha* and the name was partially retained by the 18th-century Swedish physician Linnaeus in *C. oxyacantha*. The first written record of Hawthorn may be by Petrus de Crescentis, who used it for gout in 1305.

In 1695 an anonymous healer – a woman practitioner – used the berries to treat someone showing the symptoms of hypertension.

In Europe many botanical texts first recorded Hawthorn in the 15th century. Dr. Leclerc Green has stated that the use of Hawthorn for heart conditions dates back to the 17th century. An unnamed Irish doctor is known to have used it secretly in the late 19th century to treat heart ailments. It was only after his death in 1894 that his secret was revealed by his daughter.

In the 19th century in Lorraine, France, an infusion of Hawthorn flowers was used for insomnia and palpitations. The first article about the herb appeared in 1896.

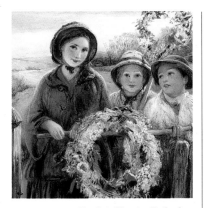

ABOVE *People in Victorian England believed that Hawthorn leaves helped those who were sworn to chastity.*

Hawthorn faded from use in the 1930s, although herbalists continued to prescribe it.

Hawthorn is documented as a useful diuretic, to treat kidney and bladder stones, and dropsy. The astringent berries were effective in cases of diarrhea, and a decoction of the flowers and berries was said to be a cure for sore throats.

Hawthorn was also used in the treatment of a wide variety of other disorders including gout, fever, pleurisy, hypertension, nervous tension, insomnia, and depression. Before recent scientific findings proved it to be a fine cardiac herb, it was always considered to be a "digestive."

GLASTONBURY HAWTHORN

The "Glastonbury Hawthorn" is a type of Hawthorn found in parts of Palestine and England. The tree is said to have been brought to England by Joseph of Arimathea. In his pilgrimage to spread the word of God he carried a staff made from Hawthorn, which he had acquired in Palestine. He is said to have visited Glastonbury in Somerset, England. Weary from traveling, he rested on "Weary-all Hill" (now called "Worral Hill"). He stuck the staff in the ground where it took root and grew into a tree. A church was later erected on the spot, now Glastonbury Abbey. The tree was regarded as sacred and was reputed only to blossom on Christmas Day (January 6, which was the day of Christ's birth before the Gregorian calendar was officially adopted). Although Hawthorn trees can still be found in the Abbey, it is believed that the original tree was cut down during the English Civil War in the mid-17th century.

BELOW *The ruins of Glastonbury Abbey, site of the "Glastonbury Hawthorn."*

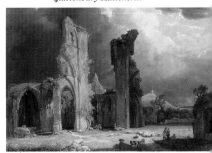

Anatomy of Hawthorn

THIS BUSHY, DENSE, *and thorny shrub grows to about 25–30ft (7.6–9m) high. It has clouds of strangely fragrant, white-pink or red blossom in May, and subsequently red berries in the fall. Its vernal green leaves turn darker and are shed by the first frosts.*

Hawthorn belongs to the *Rosaceae* family, which is made up of a large group of plants, deciduous shrubs, and trees usually bearing sharp spines.

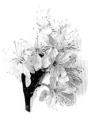

LEAVES

The leaves tend to be toothed and may also be lobed, and most species have two leafy bracts where their stalks meet the twig.

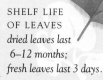

RIGHT **Hawthorn is deciduous, shedding its leaves in the fall.**

SHELF LIFE OF LEAVES
dried leaves last 6–12 months; fresh leaves last 3 days.

FLOWERS

The flowers of all Hawthorn species contain both sexes and are generally produced in clusters. They bloom in May and the blossom is made up of five-petaled flowers arranged in bunches or "corymbs" on a long stalk, each with prominent stamens, nectary, and carpels. Blossom is usually white, but can be red or pink. The overall effect of a Hawthorn tree in blossom is that of a mass of tiny rose blooms.

SHELF LIFE OF FLOWERS
dried flowers last 6–12 months; fresh flowers last 3 days.

BERRIES

The berries are greenish-red when they first appear in September, turning bright red and finally a purple red in October and November.

Hawthorn berries comprise meaty white flesh with one or two large pits in the center.

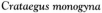

LEFT *Berry hues vary with the season.*

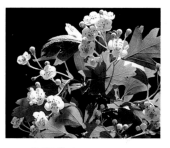

ABOVE **Crataegus monogyna** *can grow to 33ft (10m).*

Crataegus monogyna

The leaves are dark green, wedge-shaped, toothed, and deeply lobed. The strong-smelling white flowers are arranged in dense clusters, and the red fruit is barrel-shaped. This particular species is less tolerant of shade than other types of Hawthorn.

Crataegus laevigata

This shrub grows to about 20ft (6m) in height. It has fewer thorns than C. *monogyna*. The fruits are oval, about ¼–¾in (0.6–2cm) long, and contain two or three seeds. The leaves are less lobed than C. *monogyna*.

Chemical constituents

Hawthorn contains flavonoids, including oligomeric procyanidins called vitexin, quercetin, hyperoside, and rutin. These regulate the herb's cardiac actions.

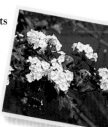

ABOVE *The flowers of* C. laevigata *are ¼–¼in (0.6cm) across.*

Other constituents are cardiotonic amines, pectin, phenolic acids including crategolic acid, citric acid, chlorogenic acid, tartaric acid, and tannins, triterpene acids, triterpenoids, and coumarins.

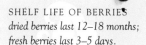

Hawthorn in action

HAWTHORN'S WIDE-RANGING *chemistry affects the body in many ways. Research scientists have found that it is able to inhibit natural enzyme responses in the blood vessels.*

HOW HAWTHORN AFFECTS THE BODY

These "angiotensin converting enzymes" (ACES) are responsible for constricting blood vessels, which help to move the blood along efficiently. The various chemical compounds of Hawthorn override these enzymes and keep the blood vessels open, thus improving circulation. This is vital in a situation where blood vessels lack tone and have

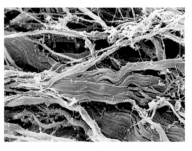

ABOVE **Collagen fiber supports the blood vessels. Hawthorn helps to rebuild collagen.**

become inert because they are clogged up with fat and calcium deposits. In this situation, an enzyme that "shuts down" the blood vessels further and restricts what little available space there is will contribute to a dangerous situation.

Hawthorn helps to lessen pain in the heart and adjacent areas, and increases warmth in cold hands and feet where the drop in temperature is due to poor circulation.

Other chemical components help to re-elasticate the blood vessel walls, and in turn assist their peristaltic and flexing action, thus promoting good blood flow and circulation throughout the entire body. The plant chemical rutin, which is a flavonoid, is partly responsible for this, and also helps to rebuild the collagen fibers that maintain the outer layers of the vessels.

HAWTHORN THE HEALER

Hawthorn's particular affinity with the heart and circulatory system provides benefits throughout the body.

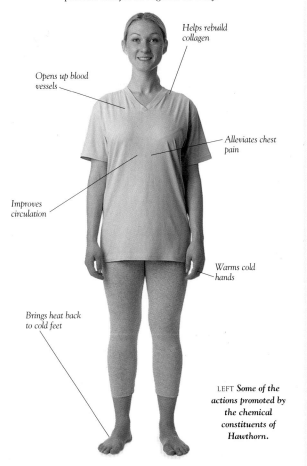

Helps rebuild collagen

Opens up blood vessels

Alleviates chest pain

Improves circulation

Warms cold hands

Brings heat back to cold feet

LEFT *Some of the actions promoted by the chemical constituents of Hawthorn.*

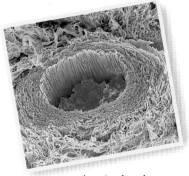

ABOVE *A section through a vein. Hawthorn helps keep veins in peak condition.*

Hawthorn's antioxidant and vitamin-C-rich chemistry assists in keeping all the circulatory components (the veins, vessels, and capillaries) young, active, and functioning properly, revitalizing, rebuilding, and helping to prevent further deterioration. Many people's physical condition does not reflect their biological age – for example, a 40-year-old can be aged 60 physiologically, simply due to the deterioration of the body. Antioxidants can help prevent and sometimes even reverse this trend. Elderly people who have naturally age-related heart weakness will also find Hawthorn beneficial. The antioxidants in the herb help to reduce inflammation, which in turn can contribute to relieving congestion, stagnation, pain, sluggishness, and associated conditions and symptoms.

The triperpene acids contained in Hawthorn can help balance low blood pressure.

Hawthorn can also play a part in lowering cholesterol levels and removing plaque that has accumulated in the arteries.

EFFECTS

❋ Normalizes and gently strengthens the contractions of the cardiac muscle.

❋ Reduces atherosclerotic plaque (fatty deposits, calcium, and other debris that block the free flow of blood).

❋ Opens up (dilates) all the blood vessels, thus improving the entire circulatory system and those organs, systems, tissues, and cells supplied with blood, potentially helping to prevent a wide range of diseases and conditions such as arteriosclerosis.

❋ Relaxes the smooth muscles of the uterus, intestines, and other areas where contractions are abnormal and constrictive and where congestion is building up.

✻ Reduces abnormal retention of water in the body, such as the bloating commonly experienced before a period.

✻ Aids digestion and the assimilation of nutrients from food and helps curb an overenthusiastic appetite.

✻ Dilates the arteries that supply the heart muscle with oxygen, blood, and fuel. The result is a more efficient heartbeat.

✻ Steadies irregular heartbeat and can be taken regularly with no side effects.

✻ Protects the heart against harmful effects of oxygen depletion – it is a powerful free-radical scavenger.

✻ Mild sedative action; this is useful in situations where stress affects the heart and vascular, digestive, and nervous systems.

✻ Helps to lower cholesterol and decreases the amount of plaque (fatty and calcium deposits) in the arteries.

✻ Aids digestion and eases sore throats and edema (see page 56).

Hawthorn works differently from other cardiac herbs: it enhances activity and nutrition by directly affecting the cells of the cardiac muscle and peripheral circulatory system. Other cardiac herbs, such as Foxglove and Lily-of-the-Valley, contain cardiac glycoside components, which have a reaction on the contractile fibers of the heart.

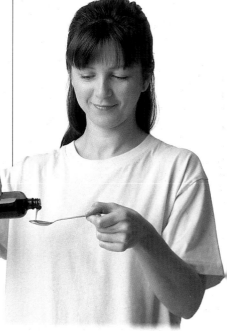

RIGHT *If you suffer from bloating before a period, Hawthorn can help.*

HAWTHORN AND THE HEART

Since the late 19th century Hawthorn has been used for various disorders of the cardiovascular system and as a heart tonic to regulate circulation. Today, Hawthorn is an official drug in the Pharmacopoeias of Brazil, China, France, Germany, Hungary, Russia, and Switzerland. As a testament to its popularity, it is an ingredient in 213 European commercial herbal formulas, designed mainly for the treatment of the heart and cardiovascular system, and sold in Europe and the United States.

Heart problems often arise out of poor dietary habits, where toxins and waste products collect and congest in the bloodstream. If a lack of exercise is coupled with this problem, then the already overly thick blood will move even less efficiently and this poor circulation further inhibits sufficient blood supply from reaching the extremities of the body. The heart and digestive organs become burdened and vital components become weakened with the strain.

Cholesterol and calcium plaque can slow the flow even further. Further problems can develop from this clogged situation, such as high or low blood pressure. The bloodstream is prevented from carrying enough basics of life – oxygen, carbon dioxide, nutrients, hormones, heat, antibodies, and enzymes – through the body.

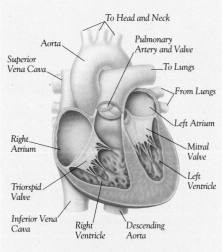

ABOVE **The two pumps of the heart squeeze blood around the body, picking up carbon dioxide and delivering oxygen.**

Hawthorn strengthens the pumping action of the heart and reduces its workload, partly by steadying the beat itself and also by increasing the heart's tolerance to oxygen deficiency. Hawthorn will normalize and gently strengthen muscle contractions of the heart, thus balancing any heart irregularities present. It does this partly by "binding" to the heart cell receptors, enabling them to use less oxygen and blood by depressing their actions. This is particularly helpful if conditions such as blocked coronary arteries or angina pectoris exist.

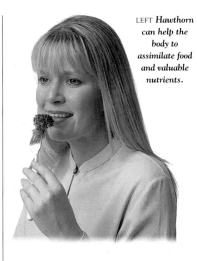

LEFT *Hawthorn can help the body to assimilate food and valuable nutrients.*

SUMMARY

Hawthorn can help treat a large number of diseases known to the medical profession. As a heart drug it can help in the treatment of heart failure, post-infarction recovery, heart valve diseases, lesions and leakages left by previous heart attacks, palpitations, angina, high and low blood pressure, heart inflammation, blood clots, angina, arteriosclerosis, old age wear-and-tear on the heart, and heart weakness following major febrile episodes.

In addition, it is valued for its ability to support the nervous system and is often used for nervous tension and insomnia. Hawthorn is a prime digestive and will help to prevent abdominal distention and poor assimilation of food; it will also assist in stabilizing nutritional levels and those diseases associated with these problems. Another area that is assisted by Hawthorn is the workings of the bladder and kidneys; it is a very safe and efficient diuretic, relieving the body of excess water in a gentle, non-exhaustive manner.

PROVEN RESULTS

When the isolated chemical components of Hawthorn were individually tested in a laboratory, their separate effects proved to be insignificant, but like so many other herbs, the rainbow of Hawthorn's chemistry, kept together as a whole, proved to be an intriguing, powerful, and very effective combination. In 1981, a four-year study of Hawthorn was commissioned by the German Ministry of Health. It was a controlled, multicenter test using clinical trials to see whether the heart function of cardiac-insufficiency patients could be improved. It was acclaimed a huge success and Hawthorn regained its old European status in the modern world as a heart herb.

Subsequently a monograph reporting these conclusions was published. It is long and detailed,

CASE STUDY: MENOPAUSE

Jessica was 50 years old and had been having heart palpitations, which were getting worse. They had begun two years earlier at the same time as her menstrual cycle became irregular and started to dwindle. Finally it became evident that she was entering the menopause. She had told her doctor about her palpitations and menopause and the doctor confirmed that they were probably connected. Jessica wanted to try a natural way of treating her heart palpitations and, after looking at various options, decided to try a tincture of Hawthorn. In just one week of taking 1 tsp (5ml) of berry and leaf tincture 3 times a day, Jessica noticed the difference and soon had her sister collecting Hawthorn leaves for her. After 3 months she switched over to Hawthorn herb tea as an alternative to the tincture and this worked equally well.

and strongly indicates that "where a loss of cardiac function" is observed, then Hawthorn is an ideal treatment. It also suggests that "where subjective feelings of congestion and oppression in the heart region" exist, then Hawthorn is a good choice, and that it is useful for easing conditions in the aging heart that do not warrant the use of digitalis (a strong heart herb that is derived from Foxglove).

WHEN TO AVOID HAWTHORN

According to the same German monograph published on Hawthorn, following four years of trials no adverse side effects were reported during the use of this remarkable herb.

Hawthorn can be used with many kinds of pharmaceutically produced drugs. However, it is suggested that it should not be combined with beta-blockers because the combination could potentially raise blood pressure.

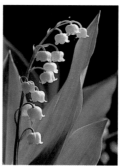

ABOVE *Avoid drugs containing Lily-of-the-Valley when taking Hawthorn.*

More important, it has been suggested that Hawthorn should not be combined with heart-drug herbs containing cardiac glycosides, such as Foxglove (which

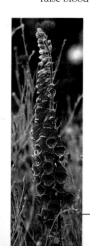

LEFT *Digitalis is a powerful drug derived from Foxglove.*

contains digitalis) and Lily-of-the-Valley (which contains convallaria). However, several studies exist where Hawthorn has been shown to increase the effectiveness of cardiac glycosides such as digitalis without increased toxicity, allowing a lower dose of the glycoside to be used. It has also been observed to date that, even with long-term medicinal use of Hawthorn, toxicity does not seem to accumulate in the body.

RESEARCH IN JAPAN

A controlled study in Japan showed that a Hawthorn berry-and-leaf combination was effective in improving symptoms of mild congestive heart failure, including poor heart function and increased blood pressure, dyspepsia, palpitations, and edema. Most patients were receiving a wide variety of pharmaceutical drugs including diuretics, cardiac glycosides, and antihypertensive agents. No adverse effects were observed on the main study group and only minor side effects were noted in the case of one particular patient.

Energy and emotion

IN AN ASTROLOGICAL CONTEXT, *Hawthorn is a masculine plant; its ruling planet and element are Mars and fire. It also has many female connections, especially in the softness of its blossom, which has been used for decorative and celebratory purposes and as a symbol of chastity and fertility for hundreds of years.*

Hawthorn flower essence:

❈ Brings hope, and instills the knowledge that your spirit is free and your body is strong.

❈ Brings balance at times of emotional stress, such as during the grieving process or when experiencing the pain of a broken relationship. It will also help with the physical stresses and strains of everyday life.

❈ Helps to promote clear thinking and recall.

❈ Encourages people to move forward in life when they need to let go of established patterns of behavior.

❈ Clears blocked emotions and helps to disperse confusion, anger, and grief.

❈ Balances inner feminine energy and sexuality.

❈ Improves the function of the immune system.

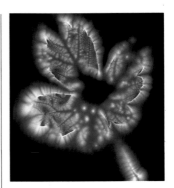

ABOVE **Kirlian photography reveals the spirit energy of a plant.**

DEALING WITH GRIEF

Crataegus monogyna brings hope and protects the body, mind, and spirit in times of grief or sadness. It instills the knowledge that our sorrows are not without end nor damaging, but just a natural part of life.

"My spirit is free. My body is a wise healer. My heart can bear this."

TRADITIONAL AFFIRMATION

TO MAKE A FLOWER ESSENCE

STANDARD QUANTITY

**Approx. 1½ cups (350ml) each of
spring water and brandy, and a handful of Hawthorn flowers**

1 *Choose a very quiet spot indoors – or a secluded area of the garden or sunny woodland if the weather allows.*
Submerge carefully chosen and freshly-picked Hawthorn flowers in a glass bowl containing 1½ cups (350ml) of spring water.

2 *Cover the bowl with protective cloth (freshly washed white cheesecloth).*

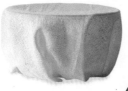

3 *Leave the bowl to stand in the sunshine for several hours – perhaps next to a window if you are indoors. If possible, try to ensure that the flowers have at least 3 hours of continuous sunshine.*

4 *After a few hours remove the flowers, using a twig to lift them out of the water. If the flowers wilt sooner than this (they may in fierce sun), then they can be removed earlier.*

5 *Measure the remaining liquid and add an equal amount of brandy. Pour into sterilized dark glass bottles; label carefully.*

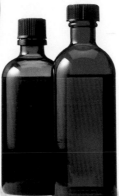

Recommended dosage

✳ *Adults: 4 drops under the tongue 4 times daily, or every half hour in times of crisis. Children: over 12 years, adult dose; 7–12 years, half adult dose; 1–7 years, quarter adult dose; younger than 1 year, consult a herbalist.*

PLANT SPIRIT ENERGIES

The spirit of the Hawthorn is different from a flower essence, which takes its power from the flowering aspect of the plant. The whole spirit of the plant enables every part of it to share its energy and properties with us.

Although its effects can be quite potent, Hawthorn is quite a subtle herb. It has the ability to give us greater refinement in how we make choices in life. The way in which some of these properties are transferred naturally leads to a greater focus of energy at the heart center.

RIGHT *The heart chakra is one of the body's energy centers, and Hawthorn has an affinity with it.*

This energy in and around the heart can be quite warming and can remain with you long after the herb has ceased being used. The spirit energy of the plant appears to have a pulsation that is close to the tempo of a heartbeat. Before taking Hawthorn, it is wise to tune in to your heartbeat for a few minutes.

Hawthorn increases your ability to "let go" of worries, and not only does this have medicinal advantages, such as letting go of stress, but also it allows you to release hurt feelings and to permit trust, both in yourself and others. Deep-seated negative thoughts can

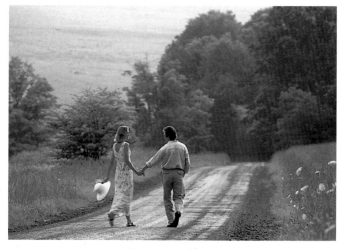

ABOVE *Your personal relationships, as well as your feelings about yourself, receive a positive boost from Hawthorn.*

be diminished or removed, and may even allow you to forgive someone about whom you may previously have had bad feelings.

To enhance this heart herb's activity, it is always good to use it alongside a meditation concentrated both on yourself and on people toward whom you have negative feelings. Although this herb facilitates love and forgiveness for others, it is, in the main, most useful for promoting self-love and self-forgiveness.

Hawthorn helps to energize the heart chakra (an energy center in the body), which naturally balances and aligns the other main chakras (see page 56). It also:

❋ Helps to release feelings of disharmony and hate.

❋ Reinstates harmony and inner tranquillity.

❋ Renews self-love and fortifies the heart.

A traditional affirmation you can use at any time to boost your self-esteem is: "My courage springs from a heart open enough to offer my strengths without self-consciousness."

Growing, harvesting, and processing

HAWTHORN GROWS EASILY *in any garden soil and will tolerate sun or partial shade. Buy a young tree from a nursery, or if you are patient, raise the plant from seed or a cutting.*

GROWING HAWTHORN

Hawthorn rarely needs to be cultivated because it will easily grow from wild seed. The seeds are usually fertilized by carrion insects, attracted by the unpleasant smell of the flowers. The aroma is similar to that of rotten meat and is produced by chemicals called triethylamines.

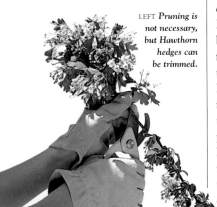

LEFT *Pruning is not necessary, but Hawthorn hedges can be trimmed.*

Homegrown If you wish to plant your own Hawthorn, you can grow it from seed or alternatively, use cuttings.

Hawthorn can be grown from seed in rich, moist soil, but it has a long period of dormancy and may take between 15 and 18 months to show its first roots. It must also be given protection from herbivores – rabbits, cows, or sheep – for the first two years. If you grow Hawthorn from seed, be aware that it will not flower for the first 20 years. If you wish to use it for hedging, grow Hawthorn in seed beds for the first two years and then transplant into rows. The young plants are ready to plant into hedges after four years. Regular weeding will help to improve their growth.

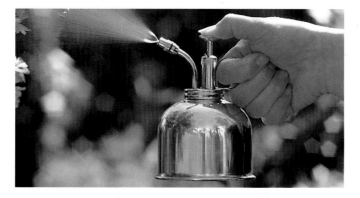

With the length of germination and the long absence of flowers while the plants mature, it may be preferable (and it is certainly easier) to grow Hawthorn from cuttings. It can be propagated this way; indeed one of its popular names "Quickset" alludes to its ability to establish itself quickly, which is a definite advantage if you are considering it for hedging. Water the plants generously, increasing both the frequency and

ABOVE *When the weather is dry, mist the leaves and water the plant well.*

quantity during the summer months. Do not let the soil dry out. Hawthorn leaves like to be misted in dry weather, but do not do it when the blossom is out.

Commercial Generally Hawthorn is not propagated specifically for commercial use; instead sites where Hawthorn has established itself tend to be claimed and used. Commercial growers of organic and "wildcrafted" plants will obtain certification for their chosen sites. Hawthorn wood has a fine grain and polishes up well. At one time it was used to make small household items, including pieces of furniture.

HAWTHORN HYBRIDS

Hawthorn hybridizes freely, so no two shrubs will look the same in a row of ancient trees or copses. Different shapes of leaves and different colored foliage and berries will all be evident, but they appear to have no detrimental effect on its medicinal qualities.

HARVESTING

The leaves should be gathered in the spring when they first unfurl (generally in April) because the young tender leaves contain the most active constituents.

ABOVE *Pick young leaves for maximum healing power.*

Flowers can usually be collected when they are in bloom in May. They are delicate, and are best used fresh; they must be dried carefully if you wish to preserve them.

The berries are collected when they have turned a deep–red color after aging on the tree, toward the end of the season. This is usually from the end of August to October. It is wonderful to collect them when they are clean and fresh just after a light late-summer rain.

Homegrown Follow the guidelines above when planning the timing of your harvest. Hawthorn has a marvelous ability to regenerate itself but you should still be careful when harvesting. When picking in the wild it is always important never to take more than a third of any plant family or colony, so that you leave plenty of flowers to go on to seed and thus perpetuate the herb.

You can harvest the leaves and flowers by pinching the base of the stalk (where it joins the woody stem) between your fingers, and twisting off the flowering top.

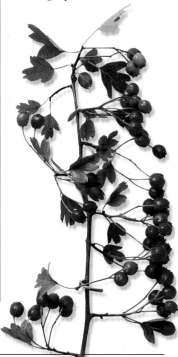

RIGHT *The berries are also known as "haws."*

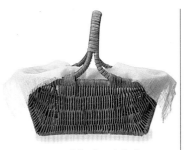

ABOVE *A lined rustic basket is practical and will protect the fragile flowers.*

The flowers are delicate, so it is helpful to have a basket lined with cheesecloth held underneath the blossoms, to ensure that no wastage occurs.

The Hawthorn berries can be harvested by using a modified apple picker, in the same way as when harvesting the flowers. However, it is not necessary to take quite as much care with this process, because the berries are robust and easy to handle.

Commercial The leaves, flowers, and berries are sometimes, but not often, harvested by using a "comb." The "comb set" is a little like a dustpan and brush, in that it has a handle and then a ragged, comblike end that gently pulls off the harvestable parts of the plant. These parts then go into the "pan" before being transferred to a collecting basket.

BELOW *Flowers are harvested in the spring, berries in the fall.*

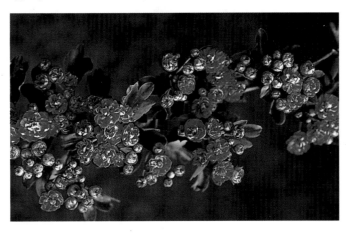

PROCESSING

The flowers, leaves, and berries should be thoroughly dried. Each part of the plant needs slightly different treatment in order to achieve the best result.

Homegrown Leaves and flowers must be dried separately because the leaves take slightly longer to dry. However, the method is the same. Put a few flowers and leaves in separate brown paper bags and hang them up in a dry place. Shake the bags frequently to make sure that enough aeration occurs.

Alternatively you can place the leaves or flowers on a wire cake rack with a layer of paper towels under them. Leave in any warm, dry place without direct sunlight, shading them if necessary. Replace the paper towels daily, until the leaves or flowers dry out.

Either method should take only a few days. Check for moisture content by placing one or two leaves or flowers in a glass jar, put on the lid and leave in the sunshine or near another heat source. If water droplets appear on the surface of the glass, then there is still a moisture content and therefore a risk of future spoilage. Should droplets form, then continue to dry the herb by repeating the drying process you have chosen.

ABOVE *Test for moisture with a sealed jar.*

Berries will take a little longer than the leaves and flowers to dry because there is more bulk and water content. Placing them in the bottom of a preheated oven is one option. Turn the oven to 480°F (250°C) and let it heat up for 30 minutes. Switch off the heat, put the berries on a baking sheet, and leave it in the bottom of the oven for 1 hour.

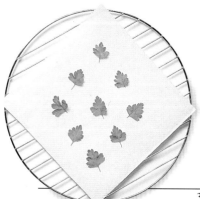

LEFT **A cake rack and paper towels make an instant drier.**

Then either switch on the heat again as low as possible for a further 2 hours, or finish the drying process in an airing cupboard. When you feel the berries may be dry (they should appear slightly wrinkled), test in a glass jar as before.

When dried, place leaves, flowers, and berries in dark storage jars with a good vacuum seal or simply a screw top.

You can also store the leaves in a brown paper bag inside a plastic bag to keep their vitality locked in.

Commercial Leaves, flowers, and berries are collected without the use of mechanical machinery. In China, Hungary, and France, initially the process is the same: the leaves, flowers, and berries are placed on commercial drying racks made from a wooden frame with nylon or cotton gauze stretched across. They are shaded from fierce sunshine and turned twice daily. In some countries sunshine may not be available in the necessary quantities in the spring or fall, so commercial

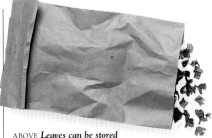

ABOVE *Leaves can be stored in a brown paper bag inserted into a plastic bag.*

blowdryers are used in a drying shed or barn. The flowers, being very light and delicate, will dry very quickly and care must be taken not to overdry them. Leaves take just a little longer and berries need longest of all. The berries are very juicy and it is vital to remove completely all the water they contain.

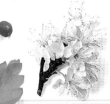

LEFT *Plant parts must be dried with care in order to retain potency.*

NOTE

In South Australia, Hawthorn has been declared a noxious weed because of its ability to proliferate so rapidly, taking over land used by other plants.

Preparations for internal use

HAWTHORN BERRIES HAVE only been used medicinally over the last few decades. Recent research has proved again what the old herbal texts stated: that there is also a great deal of valuable chemistry to be found in the leaves and flowers. Qualified modern herbalists make use of all three.

LEFT *Leaves, berries, and flowers are medicinal.*

TRIPLE HAWTHORN TINCTURE

This is a useful method of storing and taking both the fresh and dried herb. The alcohol in a tincture preserves the ingredients indefinitely, with no deterioration. Tinctures are made by soaking the leaves, blossoms, or berries (or all three) in alcohol. The alcohol will kill any unfriendly bacteria and fungal spores. The healing properties are best extracted by a mixture of water

RIGHT *Triple Hawthorn tincture.*

TINCTURES AND THE PHASES OF THE MOON

Some herbalists like to plan the making of tinctures around the moon phases, using the gravitational waxing and waning of the moon to add power and energy just like the old herb alchemists did. To do this, start the process when the moon is new, then strain and bottle at the full moon.

and alcohol (see opposite), because the flavonoids extract particularly well in water, while the other chemical constituents release their components more favorably in alcohol.

TO MAKE A TINCTURE

STANDARD QUANTITY

Use 8oz (225g) of dried Hawthorn berries, leaves, or flowers, or a mixture of all three. If you are using fresh Hawthorn, you will need a total amount of 11oz (310g). As with dried Hawthorn, you can make the tincture using only one part of the fresh shrub – berries, leaves, or flowers – or a mixture of all three. Use enough vodka and water mixture to cover – minimum 4 cups (1 liter).

1 *Place the fresh or dried leaves, flowers, and/or berries in a food processor or blender and cover with vodka; standard 45% proof is effective, but 70–80% proof is even better.*

2 *Blend the ingredients until smooth. The mixture will be particularly stiff and hard if using the berries, making it difficult for the blades to turn, and more vodka will be required in order to break them down. Work speedily when using the berries because they take only minutes to turn sticky and gluelike, because of the pectin they contain, and can set solid within 30 minutes. There is no pectin in the flowers and leaves, so there is no need to hurry if using these.*

3 *Pour the tincture into a large, sterilized, dark glass jar and cover with an airtight lid.*

4 *Shake the jar well. Label it carefully, then store it in a cool place, out of direct sunlight.*

5 *After two days, measure the contents and add water. For dried berries, leaves, and flowers, the amount of water is 20% of the volume of vodka if using 45% proof vodka, and 50–60% more water if using 70–80% proof vodka. For fresh berries, leaves, and flowers, which already have a higher water content, add half the amount of water irrespective of the strength of vodka used. Leave for at least 2 weeks but no longer than 4 weeks.*

6 *Strain the tincture through a jelly bag, preferably overnight.*

7 *Pour the liquid into dark jars; label, and store in a cool, dark place. For personal use, decant into a 2fl oz (50ml) tincture bottle. For dosages, see page 36.*

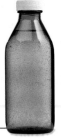

CASE STUDY: PLAQUING

Susan had arrhythmia and very cold hands and feet. She had been informed a few years earlier that she had quite bad plaquing – a build-up of fats and calcium in the arteries and veins of her bloodstream. She had also been advised that Hawthorn would help to break down the deposits that had accumulated.

However, after a year of taking a herbal formula with Hawthorn as a component, her condition seemed no better. Upon further advice she increased these doses and therefore the amount of Hawthorn. She also took Hawthorn on its own as well as the original formula.

After just one week of taking 1 tsp (5ml) three times a day of a strong Hawthorn tincture, she could for the first time feel a marked improvement. She marveled at the quick change and was pleased to think that what she felt was surely being reflected internally with reduced plaquing levels.

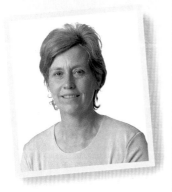

RECOMMENDED DOSAGE FOR TINCTURES FROM BERRIES, LEAVES, AND FLOWERS

❊ **Everyday and long-term use** *Adults can take 1 tsp (5ml) of tincture diluted in 5 tsp (25ml) of water 2–3 times daily.*

❊ **Acute conditions** *Adults should increase the dose frequency to every half hour until the severe symptoms have subsided.*

❊ **Children's dosages** *Over 12 years, adult dose; 7–12 years, half adult dose; 3–7 years, quarter adult dose; younger than 3 years, 2–5 drops twice daily.*

REMOVING THE ALCOHOL FROM THE TINCTURE

You may wish to avoid the small amount of alcohol in the tincture, especially if you are diabetic or expecting a baby. If this is the case, add a little boiling water to the dose you have measured out and let it stand for 5 minutes. After this time you will find that 98.5% of the alcohol has evaporated.

To dispense with alcohol completely when making the tincture, you can substitute apple cider vinegar for the vodka (use the same quantity).

HAWTHORN DECOCTION

Water-based processes preserve all the qualities of Hawthorn berries very efficiently. Dried or fresh berries may be used, although fresh berries are always best.

Making a decoction involves simmering the berries in water for a while, then straining off the liquid. This fluid will keep in the refrigerator for up to three days. Decoctions are generally used for the harder parts of plants, such as berries and roots.

TO MAKE A DECOCTION

STANDARD QUANTITY

¼oz (7g) of dried or 1½oz (40g) fresh berries to 3¾ cups (900ml) of cold water, reduced to about 2 cups (500ml) of liquid after simmering

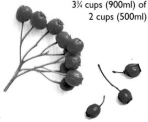

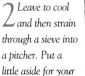

1 Put the berries and water in a saucepan (a double boiler is ideal). Bring to a boil for a few minutes, then simmer on a very low heat for about 20–30 minutes. During this time the liquid should reduce by about one third and will be quite thick due to the pectin content.

2 Leave to cool and then strain through a sieve into a pitcher. Put a little aside for your first cup. Put the pitcher in a cool place, or in the refrigerator if storing for longer than a day. If time is limited, strain off the mixture while it is still hot, straight into a thermos bottle. Have a cup immediately, then drink the rest as needed.

Recommended dosage

Adults: 2–3 cups (500–750ml) daily. Children: over 12 years, adult dose; 7–12 years, half adult dose; 3–7 years, quarter adult dose; younger than 3 years, a few sips at a time, up to a total amount of 6 tsp (30ml) a day.

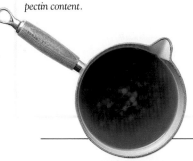

HAWTHORN INFUSION

Teas, or infusions, are usually made from the delicate parts of a plant. In the case of Hawthorn the young spring leaves and May flowers are used. With both the infusion and the decoction, adults should aim to consume 2–3 cups (500–750ml) per day. If you have not got a tea sock, this tea can also be made in a special teapot infuser, or in a coffee pot with a plunger.

TO MAKE AN INFUSION

STANDARD QUANTITY

1 tsp (2–3g) dried herb or 2 tsp (4–6g) fresh herb to 1 cup (250ml) of water, or 1oz (25g) dried herb or 1¼oz (35g) fresh herb to 2 cups (500ml) of water

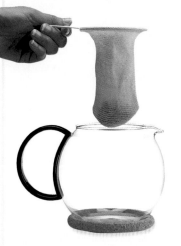

2 *Remove the tea sock and, if liked, add ½ tsp (2.5ml) of organic cold-pressed honey to sweeten. However, herbal teas are usually most effective drunk without added sweetness. Hawthorn blossom in particular has a very delicate and pleasant taste of its own.*

Recommended dosage
Adults and children should take the same doses as for a decoction (see page 37).

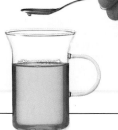

1 *Put the herb in a tea sock and place in a cup or teapot. Pour on boiling water and let stand for 7–10 minutes.*

HAWTHORN CAPSULES

Capsules can be made up from the powdered, dried berries, leaves, and flowers, and, like tinctures, they can be prepared beforehand and stored ready for use. Capsules are an easily portable remedy. Many people take commercially prepared ones containing 80–300mg of the standardized herbal extract (in capsules or tablets) two or three times a day. These standardized extracts usually have 2.2% of total flavonoid (bioflavonoid) content or about 18.75% of oligomeric procyanidins (see page 57).

ABOVE *Capsules are quickly made; an easy way of taking the herb.*

TO MAKE CAPSULES

STANDARD QUANTITY

Approximately 250–350mg of powdered herb fits into a size 00 capsule. Gelatin-free capsules for vegetarians are also available

1 *Put a little dried, finely powdered Hawthorn in a saucer and open the ends of a capsule.*

2 *Using the capsule ends as shovels, push them together until each end is full (one end will have more herb than the other).*

3 *Slide the ends together carefully, so that you do not lose any powder.*

Recommended dosage *Adults: 2 capsules 2–4 times a day. Children: over 12 years, adult dose; 7–12 years, 1 capsule 2–4 times daily; 5–7 years, 1 capsule 1–2 times daily; do not give to children younger than 5.*

RIGHT **Buy commercially prepared powdered Hawthorn (leaves, berries, and flowers).**

HAWTHORN WINE

The wine is made by first preparing a Hawthorn tea from leaves or flowers (see page 38), or a decoction from berries (see page 37). It is also possible to use these together. Sugar or honey is then dissolved in the liquid and it is left to cool. Next live yeast culture is added, which causes the liquid to ferment slowly. After several weeks, the fermentation will be complete, and the brew can be strained, bottled, and stored.

HAWTHORN ADDED TO REGULAR JUICES

If you are familiar with making your own fruit and vegetable juices and have a machine to process them, then it is useful to know that you can add fresh or dried Hawthorn berries to whatever you are juicing.
A good blood-building and heart tonic formula rich in antioxidants could be
1 part apples, ½ part Hawthorn berries, and ½ part beets. Remember that the pectin content of the berries is high and that you must consume the resultant drink immediately after you have finished juicing.

HAWTHORN LIQUEUR

A delicious liqueur can be made from Hawthorn berries and brandy. The procedure is very similar to the method for making a tincture (see page 35). Use only Hawthorn berries for making the liqueur, not leaves or flowers, and replace the vodka with brandy. Use the same proportion of alcohol/water mixture as specified for making the tincture. Pour it into a food processor and then add small amounts of (preferably fresh) berries at a time, but do not let the mixture become stiff. It should be easy to pour and not too thick so that you can strain it easily through a jelly bag or wine press.

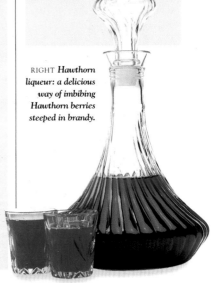

RIGHT *Hawthorn liqueur: a delicious way of imbibing Hawthorn berries steeped in brandy.*

TO MAKE HAWTHORN WINE

STANDARD QUANTITY

5–9 pints (2.25–4.5 liters) of Hawthorn berry decoction, or leaf and flower tea
3–5lb (1.5–2.5kg) of organic sugar
1 sachet of wine-making yeast
(follow instructions on pack before adding to mixture)

1 Mix the tea with the sugar by warming the tea in a saucepan and then stirring in the sugar until it is completely dissolved.

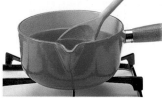

2 Switch off the heat, let cool to a temperature of approximately 65°F (18°C), and then add a live yeast culture.

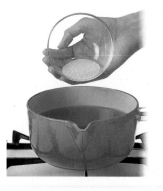

3 Let it ferment in a wine demijohn with a suitable neck lock so that carbon dioxide can escape freely. While fermentation is taking place, the demijohn should be left in a warm but shaded area.

4 Leave to ferment for up to 6 weeks. The process is complete when bubbles have stopped rippling through the brew and all the sugars have been utilized. It is important to complete the fermentation process, because hurried and incomplete fermentation will produce an unpleasant wine. Upon completion of the process, use a jelly-making strainer to strain the wine.

5 Bottle the wine, label clearly, and store in cool conditions. Remember that cleanliness when making wine is of paramount importance because any contamination can result in a spoiled brew.

NO-COOK HEDGEROW JAM

This jam is not made in the traditional manner – it requires no cooking. However, the result is surprisingly delicious and tastes very like a cooked jam. It has a delightful flavor and good consistency. It is also very nutritious, retaining its rich array of beneficial vitamins and healthy flavonoids.

TO MAKE HEDGEROW JAM

STANDARD QUANTITY

2 parts Hawthorn berries, 2 parts Blackberries
2 parts Elderberries, ½ part Rosehips
enough pure vegetable glycerine to cover the berries

1 Pick over all the berries to remove any that are damaged, taking care with the crushable Blackberries and Elderberries.

2 Weigh out the correct quantities. It is important to measure accurately for two reasons: the water content of the Elderberries and Blackberries balances the thickness and sweetness of the glycerine, and the relatively small quantity of Rosehips is because their fluffy seeds would spoil the jam's texture if a larger amount were used.

3 Place all the berries in a blender and just cover with vegetable glycerine. Alternatively, you can cover them with half glycerine and half maple syrup mixture.

You will probably find that it is difficult for the blades to turn, but persist and add more watery berries rather than more glycerine or maple syrup, to avoid making the jam too sweet. The mixture will thicken very quickly, so you will need to work fast.

4 When the mixture is fairly smooth, transfer it to sterilized glass jars. Seal them and label clearly with the contents and the date. The jam will last for up to a year unopened in the refrigerator. Once the jar is opened, however, you should use the jam within 2 weeks.

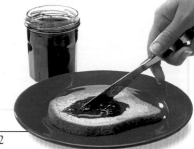

TO MAKE MEDICINAL HAWTHORN SYRUP

STANDARD QUANTITY

As a rough guide, use 2½lb (1.1kg) of dried, crushed berries with enough spring water to cover them. You can also use smaller quantities of berries and water.

1 Soak the dried and crushed Hawthorn berries in spring water for 1–2 days. Use enough water to cover the berries by 1in (2.5cm).

2 Process the mixture in a blender or wrap the berries in cheesecloth and crush them once again with a hammer. Leave to soak for another day

3 Boil for 2 minutes over a medium heat, then reduce the heat and simmer for 30 minutes. Finally, switch off the heat and let steep for 30 minutes.

4 Strain the mixture thoroughly, reserve the fluid, and refrigerate the liquid when cool. If necessary, squeeze the juice through a fine but strong cheesecloth bag. It is important to extract as much of the juice as you can. A wine press is ideal for this hard job.

5 Now measure the total volume of all the simmered and strained berry water. Simmer again on a low heat until it reduces down to one quarter of the original volume.

6 Measure the liquid, then mix it with an equal amount of brandy (the best you can afford) and vegetable glycerine mixture. The mixture should be half brandy and half vegetable glycerine. Pour into sterilized bottles and refrigerate. It keeps indefinitely.

Recommended dosage Adults: 6–12 tbsp (90–180ml) a day. Children: over 12 years, adult dose; 7–12 years, half adult dose; 3–7 years, quarter adult dose; younger than 3, 1–3 tsp (5–15ml) in total per day.

NOTE

American herbalist Dr. Richard Schulze uses Hawthorn syrup as a base for a much more powerful heart tonic: 8 parts Hawthorn berry syrup, 1 part Motherwort tincture, 1 part Ginger root tincture, 1 part Cactus grandiflorus tincture, and 1 part Cayenne tincture. Recommended dosage for adults: 1 tsp (5ml) 3–8 times a day.

Natural medicine for everyone

HAWTHORN IS CONSIDERED *by the qualified herbalists who prescribe it as extremely safe to take both in the long term and the short term. The British herbalist Simon Mills refers to Hawthorn as one of the safest plants available. Other practitioners refer to it as a "heart food."*

PREGNANCY

High blood pressure, irregular heartbeat, varicose veins, and thrombosis can sometimes accompany pregnancy; Hawthorn can safely support the mother in these situations, without causing any harm to the growing baby. However, small doses are always advisable. Dr. John Christopher, who practiced herbal medicine for more than 50 years in the United States, prescribed a combination of Hawthorn, Garlic, Cayenne, and cucumber for high blood pressure.

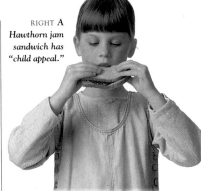

RIGHT **A Hawthorn jam sandwich has "child appeal."**

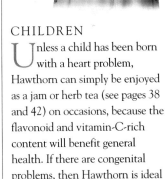

LEFT *Garlic, Cayenne, grated cucumber, and Hawthorn.*

CHILDREN

Unless a child has been born with a heart problem, Hawthorn can simply be enjoyed as a jam or herb tea (see pages 38 and 42) on occasions, because the flavonoid and vitamin-C-rich content will benefit general health. If there are congenital problems, then Hawthorn is ideal to help repair, and protect against a wide variety of conditions, such as high inherited levels of cholesterol. In the UK a greater number of children are being born with heart-related problems, or developing them younger and younger. In the past, certain heart conditions seen by doctors and surgeons in patients over 40 years of age are now being seen in 20-year-olds, due largely to poor nutritional habits. Many children's diets today are far less nutritious and decidedly more harmful in content than those provided in earlier times, even when compared to the diets of underprivileged children in, for example, 19th-century Europe. In North America, however, some diet strategies are starting to reverse heart problems.

ELDERLY PEOPLE

Hawthorn is one herb that everybody over 50 years old should use daily or weekly. It is an ideal treatment for people who become breathless when walking and who cannot bend down, for those with breathing problems, angina pains, or experience of heart episodes (heart attacks).

The herb's qualities as an excellent digestive are also valuable: this can be a tricky area as we age. Hawthorn can safely be mixed with many drugs already being taken on a daily basis. However, there should be caution when heart drugs based on cardiac glycosides, for example digitalis, are being taken. The same can be said of beta-blockers.

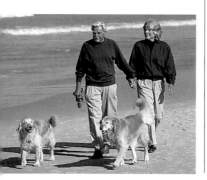

LEFT *If you become breathless when walking, Hawthorn can help to ease the problem.*

CAUTION

Always consult a qualified herbalist or medical practitioner before embarking on any treatment for a serious illness, or if you are considering using other heart drugs or beta-blockers.

Herbal combinations

HERBAL COMBINATIONS ARE *used where the effect of a single herb needs to be complemented in a particular way. However, if you are pregnant, breastfeeding, or have a serious medical condition, you should consult a qualified herbal practitioner before trying any of the following formulas, because some of the herbs may be unsuitable for you to take.*

Many herbal formulas consist of one main herb and others to support it in varying proportions. A formula may change over time to reflect the changing state of the disease or imbalance. Some heart herbs have varying amounts of cardiac glycosides, which strongly stimulate the heart. These must only be prescribed by a qualified medical practitioner and have therefore not been listed here.

CHILBLAINS

When poor circulation causes cold hands and feet, chilblains can develop. These are areas of skin that have become so tight and contracted due to the cold that they are deprived both of blood and oxygen. Itching, swelling, and a burning sensation will result.

Formula 3 parts Hawthorn berries, flowers, and leaves; 1 part Prickly Ash berries and bark; 1 part Ginger rhizome; ¼ part Cayenne pods (all strong circulatory herbs).

ABOVE **Prickly Ash berries help to clear up chilblains.**

Dosage Adults: 1 tsp (5ml) tincture 3–4 times a day. Children: over 12 years, adult dose; 7–12 years, ½ tsp (2.5ml) 3–4 times a day; the heat of Cayenne may not be palatable to children under 7 years, so consult a qualified herbalist.

HEART TONIC AND RESTORATIVE

This formula, which should be taken in tincture form, aims to tone and strengthen the heart and support the circulation.

Formula 6 parts Hawthorn berries, leaves, and flowers, 4 parts Motherwort leaves and flowers, 1 part Ginger rhizomes, ¼ part Cayenne pods (hottest variety or increase percentage).

ABOVE **Fiery Cayenne is a stimulant.**

Dosage Adults: 1 tsp (5ml) 3–4 times a day. Children: over 12 years, adult dose; 7–12 years ½ tsp (2.5ml) 3–4 times daily; 3–7 years, ¼ tsp (1.25ml) 3 times daily; younger than 3, consult a qualified herbalist.

RIGHT **Motherwort is a heart tonic and muscle relaxant, helping to treat palpitations.**

Hawthorn is a fine, all-round cardiovascular restorative that will help normalize not only heart function but also that of the entire circulatory system. The herb works both in the short term and long term.

ABOVE **Ginger is warming; good for circulation.**

Motherwort is a relaxing nervine: that is, it favorably affects the nervous system, helping to dissolve tension and anxiety and at the same time acting as a general tonic for the heart. Where the heartbeat is too fast, perhaps caused by tension and anxiety, this herb will help immediately. Ginger and Cayenne both serve to contribute an extra beneficial effect to the circulatory system.

ATHEROMA AND ARTERIOSCLEROSIS FORMULA

This tincture formula is ideal for any condition that causes thick, fatty, cholesterol-saturated blood. It will help thin the blood, open the blood vessels, and reduce the stickiness of the blood components, while assisting in removing fat deposits.

Formula

4 parts Red Clover flowers and leaf tops, 4 parts Hawthorn blossoms, leaves, and berries, 4 parts Lime blossom flowers, 3 parts Burdock root, 3 parts Ginkgo leaves, 2 parts Alfalfa leaves, 2 parts Garlic syrup (see page 43), 1 part Cayenne pods.

ABOVE *Red clover is rich in coumarins, which will thin the blood.*

Dosage

Adults: 1 tsp (5ml) 3–4 times daily. Children: over 12 years, adult dose; 5–12 years, half adult dose; younger than 5 years, consult a qualified medical practitioner.

Lime blossom helps to remove cholesterol and prevent future build-ups.

Red clover and Alfalfa thin the blood, and Garlic is rich in sulfurous compounds that beneficially affect blood cholesterol and regulate triglyceride levels. Cayenne stimulates the peripheral circulation, helps thin the blood and disperses fatty deposits. Ginkgo prevents the blood from becoming sticky.

ABOVE *Lime blossom helps to reduce high blood pressure.*

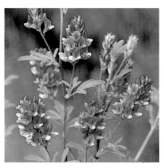

ABOVE *Alfalfa cleans the veins and arteries, removing any obstructions.*

NOTE

The Garlic is in syrup form in this formula whereas the other components are tinctures. The syrup is made in much the same way as Hawthorn syrup (see page 43). If the syrup cannot be made or consumed in this way, take separately either in your food (1–3 cloves daily) or in capsules (2 capsules 3 times daily).

STRESS-BASED HEART AND CIRCULATORY WEAKNESS

Lots of heart problems are either initiated by or made much worse by anxiety and stress. There are many heart nervines and the following tincture formula can vary slightly in practice.

Formula

3 parts Skullcap leaves, 3 parts Hawthorn berries, leaves, and flowers, 2 parts Black Cohosh root, 2 parts Valerian root, 2 parts Lime Tree flowers, ¼ part Cayenne pods.

Dosage

Adults: 1 tsp (5ml) 3–4 times daily. Children: over 12 years, adult dose; 7–12 years, half adult dose; younger than 7 years, consult a qualified medical practitioner.

Skullcap deals with conditions ranging from depression to seizures. It helps renew the actual components of the nervous system: taking it over a long period of time ensures lasting renewal can take place. Black Cohosh is a powerful relaxant and normalizer of nerve impulses.

ABOVE *One of the many members of the skullcap family.*

CASE STUDY: HEART DAMAGE

Jack Dobson was just 37 years old but he had already had two heart episodes (heart attacks), one minor and a slightly more severe one just a year later. The last episode showed a little bit of scar damage on the heart itself. Jack was determined to improve his lifestyle, and taking Hawthorn was part of his new health regime. He had heard that Hawthorn could minimize damage to the heart in the event of a heart episode and would also lessen the likelihood of another episode over the long term, while at the same time improving overall well-being.

Four years later Jack still takes 1 tsp (5ml) of Hawthorn tincture in the morning and 1 cup of Hawthorn tea in the evening. He feels much fitter and no longer has heart pains or any feeling that he is at risk of another episode.

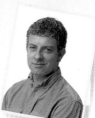

Valerian works similarly to Black Cohosh, but it is particularly helpful if sleep is difficult. Lime Tree flowers calm the nervous system and treat high blood pressure and arteriosclerosis, by helping the veins and arteries function more efficiently. Cayenne helps the circulation.

POOR MEMORY

This formula, taken as a tincture, will help to clarify the thought processes and improve the memory, particularly useful for old people but also helpful to the young.

Formula

Equal parts of Ginkgo leaves, Hawthorn berries and flowers, Prickly Ash bark and berries.

Dosage Adults: 1 tsp (5ml) 3–4 times daily. Children: over 12 years, adult dose; 7–12 years, ½ tsp (2.5ml) 3–4 times daily; 3–7 years, ¼ tsp (1.25ml) 3 times daily; younger than 3 years, consult a qualified medical practitioner. Ginkgo is a cardiovascular herb, like Hawthorn. It can thin sticky blood, guard against blood clots, and very

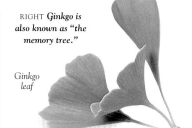

RIGHT *Ginkgo is also known as "the memory tree."*

Ginkgo leaf

strongly improve cerebral circulation, aiding memory and concentration. For this reason it is also used in the treatment of early senile dementia. Hawthorn will support Ginkgo in this work.

Prickly Ash encourages forceful blood circulation, providing almost instantaneous blood surges to the brain.

BELOW *If your child is finding school a struggle, this formula may help.*

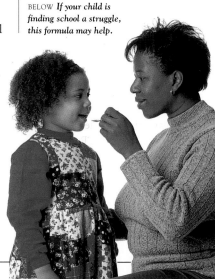

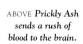

Prickly Ash bark

ABOVE *Prickly Ash sends a rush of blood to the brain.*

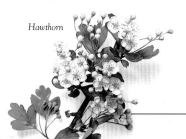

Hawthorn

VARICOSE VEINS

Personal genetics and constitution, a lifestyle in which lack of exercise is combined with long hours of standing, or even pregnancy are all factors that can cause poor circulation, which in turn can result in varicose veins. Veins become "varicose" when they become enlarged, swollen, and sometimes twisted. They can occur at any age and anywhere in the body, but they are generally associated with the legs. The herbs chosen in this tincture formula are able to stimulate peripheral circulation and therefore encourage adequate blood flow to the legs.

Formula

3 parts Hawthorn leaves, flowers, and berries, 3 parts Prickly Ash bark and berries, 3 parts Horse chestnut, 1 or 2 parts Dandelion root, ½ part Ginger rhizome, ¼ part Cayenne pods.

Dosage Adults: 1 tsp (5ml) 3–4 times daily.

LEFT *Hawthorn and regular exercise can help to prevent varicose veins.*

Hawthorn opens up the arteries and veins and enables better circulation. Prickly Ash, Cayenne, and Ginger are also strong circulatory herbs and will tackle the problem very quickly. Horse chestnut will strengthen the blood vessels – which is important because they will be weak and will need to bear the force of the increased and vital circulation.

The Dandelion is included in case there is also water retention; if there is not it will not unduly force the kidneys, but it is optional and can be removed from the formula if it seems unnecessary.

Cayenne

Dandelion root

RIGHT *Herbs to boost circulation and inhibit water retention.*

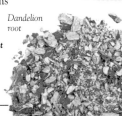

Conditions chart

THIS CHART *is a guide to some of the ailments that Hawthorn can help to treat (see pages 34–43 for dosages), but it is not intended to replace other forms of treatment. Always consult your doctor or another qualified medical practitioner before embarking on a course of treatment.*

NAME	INTERNAL USE
ANGINA PECTORIS	Tincture, capsules, syrup
ARRHYTHMIA	Tincture, decoction, syrup
ARTERIOSCLEROSIS	Tincture, decoction, syrup
ARTHRITIS	Tincture, decoction, capsules
BLOOD PRESSURE (BALANCES)	Tincture, decoction, syrup
CHILBLAINS	Tincture, decoction, wine
CIRCULATION (IMPROVES)	Tincture, infusion, wine
COLD (STOPS YOU FROM FEELING COLD)	Tincture, decoction, syrup, liqueur

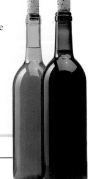

NAME	INTERNAL USE
FLUID RETENTION	Tincture, decoction, syrup
HEART PALPITATIONS	Tincture, decoction, syrup
HEART WEAKNESS	Tincture, decoction, syrup
HEMORRHOIDS	Tincture, decoction, capsules
MILD MITRAL STENOSIS	Tincture, decoction, syrup
PHLEBITIS	Tincture, decoction, capsules
SORE THROAT	Infusion, decoction, syrup
VARICOSE ULCERS	Tincture, decoction, syrup
VARICOSE VEINS	Tincture, decoction, syrup, capsules

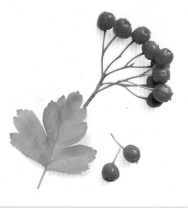

How Hawthorn works

HAWTHORN IS COMPOSED of a wide range of exciting plant chemistry that works best as a whole, allowing the "herbal synergy" to work as a team rather than as isolated components.

Hawthorn can be used either long term or short term, but do not assume it is a slow herb; it is capable of dealing with situations very quickly.

Hawthorn preparations can vary in their potency, according to how they have been made.

❧ Hawthorn's flavonoidlike complexes are responsible for the cardiac actions of the plant. They increase the use of oxygen by the heart, and help metabolize enzymes. The complexes also act as a mild dilator of blood vessels away from the heart; this lowers blood pressure and relieves the burden on the heart.

❧ Four such flavonoids (or bioflavonoids) in Hawthorn include oligomeric procyanidins called vitexin, quercetin, hyperoside, and rutin.

The flavonoids also aid the stabilization of collagen, helping to prevent and treat diseases such as atherosclerosis.

❧ Flavonoids are very potent, particularly here where they help prevent the deterioration of the

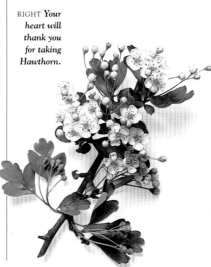

RIGHT *Your heart will thank you for taking Hawthorn.*

whole system. The walls of the blood vessels are kept elastic, flexible, dilated, strengthened, and relaxed. Cholesterol levels can be lowered and the amount of plaque in the arteries reduced.

❧ Hawthorn also contains cardiotonic amines, a nitrogen-type derivative of amino acids; they include phenylalanine and tyramine, which are believed to help with all manner of cardiac balancing effects, for example promoting better circulation, and lowering high blood pressure.

❧ Pectin also occurs in large quantities in Hawthorn (it makes a solid jelly minutes after the berries are liquefied). Pectin is known both to remove all manner of toxins, including heavy metals and radiation, and to enhance the physiological function of the digestive tract through its physical, chemical, and antibacterial properties.

❧ Hawthorn contains phenolic acids, including crategolic acid, citric acid, chlorogenic acid, tartaric acid, and triterpene acids, the last of which increase coronary blood flow. Citric acid is cleansing and cooling, having an alkalizing and acid-balancing effect on the body; it also stimulates bile production and assists in good digestion. Foods that create a sick body are often highly acidic.

❧ Hawthorn's ability to remove water is partly explained by its tannin content, which helps promote the release of water by helping to "rigidify" and dry out cell walls. Tannin is also useful as an anti-infection agent.

❧ Hawthorn contains triterpenoids, which have anti-inflammatory, pain-killing, and oxygen-supplying effects.

❧ The blood-thinning and plaque-dissolving qualities of Hawthorn are partly due to its coumarin content (see page 56). In the plant world coumarin is prevalent in spring greens.

MAIN EFFECTS

❧ Dilates peripheral circulation and that of the heart itself.

❧ Increases the tone of the heart, slowing it down, providing oxygen, and slightly stimulating the pulse rate.

❧ Sedative effects of Hawthorn lower high blood pressure and the cardiotonic effects raise low blood pressure.

Glossary

ANGINA PECTORIS
A sudden intense pain in the chest, caused by a momentary lack of sufficient blood supply to the heart.

ANTIOXIDANTS
In current models of immunity, these substances, found particularly in high-chlorophyll foods, are understood to protect the cells from free-radicals, which themselves have been created through oxygenation.

ARRHYTHMIA
Any deviation from a normal heartbeat.

ARTERIOSCLEROSIS
Hardening of the arteries.

BETA-BLOCKERS
Drugs used in the treatment of angina, hypertension, migraine, and anxiety states.

CARDIAC GLYCOSIDES
Compounds that cause a reaction in the contractile fibers of the heart, strongly stimulating it.

CHAKRAS
In Eastern medicine, chakras are believed to be the body's energy centers. They exist along the mid-line of the body, in line with the spinal column. They are located in seven regions of the body: the base of the spine, the genitals, the abdomen, the heart, the throat, the center of the forehead, and the crown of the head.

CHOLESTEROL
A waxy, insoluble substance found in almost all body tissues. High levels of cholesterol in the blood are linked to heart disease.

COUMARINS
Substances with anticoagulation properties. They are also sedative, calming, and uplifting.

DECOCTION
A process used to prepare the tougher parts of a plant, such as berries and roots, for consumption. The plant parts are simmered in water, and the liquid is strained off for use.

EDEMA
Excessive accumulation of fluid in the body tissues.

FLAVONOIDS
Antioxidants that act on the immune system.

FREE-RADICALS
Atoms that exist for a brief period before reacting to create a stable molecule. They are capable of causing damage within the body.

IMMUNITY
The capacity and function of the body to fend off foreign bodies (fungi, viruses, bacteria), and/or disarm and eject them.

INFUSION
Infusions are water-based herbal preparations used to extract the active qualities of leaves and flowers. They are drunk as a tea.

MITRAL STENOSIS
Narrowing of the mitral valve by inflammation, nearly always caused by rheumatic fever.

OLIGOMERIC PROCYANIDINS
Flavonoids that regulate the cardiac actions of Hawthorn.

PHLEBITIS
Inflammation of a vein.

PLAQUE
In this context, plaque does not refer to the substance we try to eradicate from our teeth; however, it does have similar properties in that it is a build-up of undesirable matter – fats and calcium – in the veins and arteries.

STEROIDS
Fat-soluble organic compounds that have important physiological actions. They include sterols, for example cholesterol, bile acids, hormones, vitamin D, cardiac glycosides, and sapogenins.

TINCTURE
An alcohol and water-based preparation. It is made from various parts of a plant, in combination or individually.

TRIGLYCERIDE
A fatty-acid ester of glycerol and carboxylic acid. This is the form in which fat is stored in the body.

Further reading

ELDERS HERBAL, *David Hoffman* (Healing Arts Press, 1993)

ENCYCLOPAEDIA OF MEDICINAL PLANTS, *Andrew Chevallier* (Dorling Kindersley, 1996)

ENCYCLOPEDIA OF FLOWER REMEDIES, *C. G. Harvey and A. Cochrane* (Thorsons, 1995)

ESSENTIAL SCIENCE CHEMISTRY, *Freemantle & Tidy* (Oxford University Press, 1983)

EXCURSION FLORA OF THE BRITISH ISLES, *A.R. Clapham and E.F. Warburg* (Cambridge University Press, 1958)

HISTORY OF BRITAIN'S TREES, *Gerald Wilkinson* (Hutchinson, 1981)

MANUAL OF CONVENTIONAL MEDICINE FOR ALTERNATIVE PRACTITIONERS, *Stephen Gasgoine* (Jigame Press, 1993)

MODERN HERBAL, *Mrs. M. Grieve* (Peregrine Books, 1931)

SCHOOL OF NATURAL HEALING, *Dr. Christopher* (Christopher Publications, 1976)

SPIRITUAL PROPERTIES OF HERBS, *Gurudas* (Cassandra Press, 1988)

TEXTBOOK OF ADVANCED HERBOLOGY, *Terry Willard* (Wild Rose College of Natural Healing, 1992)

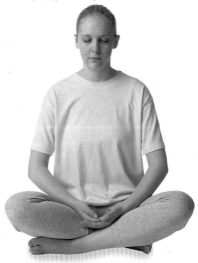

Useful addresses